YOUR KNOWLEDGE HAS VALUE

AF138324

- We will publish your bachelor's and
  master's thesis, essays and papers

- Your own eBook and book -
  sold worldwide in all relevant shops

- Earn money with each sale

Upload your text at www.GRIN.com
and publish for free

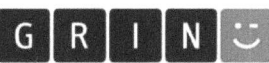

Torticollis in Focus

A Comprehensive Guide to Understanding and Treating Torticollis

Divya Shukla

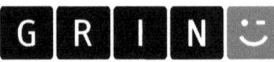

Bibliographic information published by the German National Library:

The German National Library lists this publication in the National Bibliography; detailed bibliographic data are available on the Internet at http://dnb.dnb.de.

ISBN: 9783389125151
This book is also available as an ebook.

© GRIN Publishing GmbH
Trappentreustraße 1
80339 München

All rights reserved

Print and binding: Books on Demand GmbH, Norderstedt, Germany
Printed on acid-free paper from responsible sources.

The present work has been carefully prepared. Nevertheless, authors and publishers do not incur liability for the correctness of information, notes, links and advice as well as any printing errors.

GRIN web shop: https://www.grin.com/document/1571783

TABLE OF CONTENTS

Chapter

A medical condition known as torticollis affects the manner in which the head and neck are positioned. It is distinguished by an abnormal head posture caused by the neck twisting or tilting. With a 3:2 boy-to-girl ratio and a little association with post-term birth, the average age of onset ranges from 4 to 8 weeks. Though usually spontaneous, onset can also be related to trauma, such as forceps-assisted delivery, vacuum extraction, or cervical spine injury.

About 10% of patients have a history of recent immunizations and 5% of patients have a congenital neck tumor or neck trauma. The Latin terms for "twisted" and "neck," which highlight the deviations in neck alignment, are the source of the condition's name. Estimates of the reported incidence vary greatly, ranging from 0.3% to 2.0% of live births. It's crucial to remember that underdiagnosis and misdiagnosis could mean that these estimates don't accurately reflect the condition's actual prevalence. The asymmetry linked to left torticollis is further highlighted by the fact that it occurs 3:2 more often than right.

Torticollis is caused by the abnormal contraction of neck muscles, which results in pain and a restricted range of motion. Affected persons may have profound pain and functional deficits as a result. The goals of torticollis treatment are to reduce symptoms, increase neck mobility, and encourage proper head and neck alignment. Stretching methods, postural positioning techniques, and physical therapy exercises are frequently used to treat the disease. In numerous cases, correcting structural defects that contribute to torticollis may need surgical intervention. All things considered, the best results for people with torticollis depend on early detection and suitable treatments.

Infants and early children are susceptible to a somewhat common ailment called torticollis, occasionally referred to as wry neck. It is crucial that pediatricians with all levels of training are knowledgeable in identifying, diagnosing, and starting the right treatment plans for newborns who exhibit torticollis. Despite being traditionally associated with skull structural abnormalities, congenital muscle torticollis actually makes up the majority of instances and is a contributing factor to aberrant postures. The development of secondary issues such as plagiocephaly (asymmetry of the skull), facial asymmetry, vision difficulties, and even scoliosis can result from a failure to identify and deal with this condition in a timely manner.

Despite the fact that many torticollis cases may seem harmless, it is important to remember that children with the condition may have a significant 30% to 35% decrease in their neck's range of motion, which may have long-term effects on the soft tissues and bone structures. To reduce the possible aftereffects of torticollis, early detection and therapy are therefore essential. Furthermore, it is essential to underestimate the need for continuing follow-up since managing any residual deficits and ensuring the best possible results for impacted children require ongoing tracking. Referrals to specialists may occasionally be taken into consideration as an extra choice to offer children with orthodontics complete care and expertise..

Chapter

Causes and risk factors

Numerous congenital and acquired reasons can be linked to torticollis. The most prevalent type of the disorder, congenital muscular torticollis, is frequently identified in the first six to eight weeks of life and is typified by a soft, non-tender enlargement in the s ternocleidomastoid muscle that progressively regresses over time (Hensinger & Jones, 1982). Traumatic traumas, including birth injuries or neck strains, as well as a number of underlying medical disorders like infections, are additional possible causes of torticollis.

Before exploring the causes and risk factors, it's critical to understand that there are various varieties of torticollis:

1. Congenital torticollis: a condition that develops at birth and is frequently brought on by malformed muscles or improper posture during pregnancy.

2. Acquired torticollis: This type appears later in life and may be brought on by infections, trauma, or muscle spasms.

3. Cervical dystonia, or spasmodic torticollis, is a neurological condition in which aberrant head postures are caused by involuntary muscle spasms.

Causes of Torticollis

Congenital Factors:

Muscle Abnormalities: Congenital torticollis is frequently linked to a shortening of the sternocleidomastoid muscle on one side of the neck. This muscle connects the sternum and clavicle to the mastoid process behind the ear.

Birth Trauma: Injuries during delivery, such as excessive pulling on the head or shoulder during a difficult birth, can lead to damage or tightness in neck muscles.

Neurological Conditions:

Cervical Dystonia: This neurological disorder leads to involuntary muscle contractions in the neck, causing abnormal postures.

Brain injury or stroke: Damage to areas of the brain that control movement can result in torticollis.

Infections and Inflammation:

Meningitis: inflammation of the protective membranes covering the brain and spinal cord can lead to stiffness in the neck.

Upper Respiratory Infections: These infections may cause inflammation that affects neck muscles.

Trauma or Injury:

Whiplash injuries from car accidents or falls can strain neck muscles, leading to torticollis.

Sports injuries involving sudden movements of the head may also contribute.

Musculoskeletal Disorders

Conditions like arthritis affecting cervical vertebrae can lead to pain and restricted movement, resulting in compensatory postures that resemble torticollis.

Medications and drug reactions:

Certain medications, particularly antipsychotics (e.g., haloperidol), may induce acute dystonic reactions leading to symptoms resembling torticollis.

Genetic Predisposition:

Some studies suggest a hereditary component where individuals with family histories of muscular disorders may have increased susceptibility.

Environmental Factors:

Prolonged poor posture during activities such as reading or using electronic devices may contribute over time.

Sleeping positions that place undue stress on neck muscles could also be a factor.

Psychological Factors:

Stress and anxiety have been implicated in exacerbating muscle tension, which could lead to spasmodic forms of torticollis.

Idiopathic Causes:

In many cases, especially with spasmodic torticollis, no clear cause is identified despite thorough investigation.

Risk Factors for Developing Torticollis

1. **Age Factor**:
   - Congenital torticollis typically presents at birth; however, acquired forms are more common among adults aged 30-60 years due to degenerative changes in cervical structures.
2. **Gender Disparity**:
   - Women are statistically more likely than men to develop certain types of torticollis, particularly spasmodic torticollis.
3. **Family History**:
   - A familial tendency toward musculoskeletal disorders increases risk; individuals with relatives who have experienced similar conditions should be aware of their predisposition.
4. **Occupational Hazards**:
   - Jobs requiring repetitive neck movements or prolonged static postures (e.g., desk jobs) increase susceptibility due to muscle fatigue and strain over time.
5. **Previous Neck Injuries or Conditions**:
   - Individuals with prior history of cervical spine issues are at higher risk for developing torticollis due to residual effects on muscle function and alignment.
6. **Physical Activity Levels**:
   - Sedentary lifestyles may weaken neck muscles leading them susceptible to strain when sudden movements occur; conversely, excessive physical activity without proper conditioning might also trigger episodes.

7. **Underlying Health Conditions**:
   - Pre-existing conditions such as Parkinson's disease or multiple sclerosis can predispose individuals toward developing secondary forms of torticollis due to motor control issues.
8. **Use of Certain Medications**
   - Long-term use of specific medications known for inducing dystonic reactions increases risk significantly; patients should consult healthcare providers regarding potential side effects related specifically to their prescribed treatments.
9. *Psychosocial Stressors*: - High levels of stress have been shown through various studies correlating psychological well-being with physical manifestations including tension-related disorders like spasmodic torticollis; managing stress effectively could mitigate risks associated with this condition.

In conclusion, understanding both causes and risk factors associated with torticollis provides valuable insights into prevention strategies as well as guiding effective treatment options tailored towards individual needs based upon u underlying etiologies present within each case scenario encountered clinically.

Importance of Early Intervention

Understanding Torticollis and Its Effects

Torticollis, particularly congenital muscular torticollis (CMT), is a condition characterized by the tilting of a child's head to one side due to tightness in the sternocleidomastoid muscle. If left untreated, this condition can lead to significant developmental issues, including delayed motor milestones, postural abnormalities such as scoliosis, vision problems, and social-emotional challenges. The tilted head position can interfere with a child's ability to engage in normal activities and may cause self-consciousness or difficulty interacting with peers.

Consequences of Delayed Treatment

The consequences of delaying intervention for torticollis can be severe. Research indicates that children who do not receive early treatment may experience prolonged physical therapy episodes—up to 9 to 10 months—compared to those who start therapy before 1 month of age, who often achieve normal range of motion within just 1.5 months. Delayed treatment can also lead to secondary complications such as facial asymmetries, TMJ pain, contracture formation, and even surgical interventions later in life.

Benefits of Early Intervention

Early intervention is crucial for several reasons:

1. Improved Range of Motion: Children diagnosed with CMT before 1 month of age have a 98% success rate in achieving normal cervical range of motion within approximately 1.5 months when they undergo physical therapy.
2. Reduced Treatment Duration: Starting therapy early significantly reduces the overall duration required for treatment. Infants referred at younger ages typically require fewer sessions and less intensive care compared to those referred later.
3. Enhanced Motor Skills Development: Early intervention helps children catch up on motor skills that may be delayed due to their condition. This includes important milestones like rolling over, sitting up, crawling, and walking.
4. Better Quality of Life: By addressing the physical limitations caused by torticollis early on, children are more likely to participate fully in social activities and develop healthy self-esteem.
5. Prevention of Secondary Conditions: Timely intervention helps prevent the development of associated conditions such as scoliosis or craniofacial deformities that could arise from prolonged abnormal positioning.
6. Parental Education and Support: Early intervention programs often include education for parents on how to support their child's development through daily exercises and proper positioning techniques at home.

Conclusion

In summary, early identification and intervention for torticollis are critical for optimizing outcomes in affected infants. The earlier a child receives appropriate therapy, the better their chances are for a full recovery without long-term complications.

Objectives of This Guide

- To provide an understanding of torticollis, including its origins and manifestations.
- To describe the anatomical and muscular factors involved in torticollis.
- To outline effective assessment techniques for accurate diagnosis.
- To emphasize the significance of timely intervention and management strategies.

Understanding Torticollis: Origins and Manifestations

Torticollis, also known as "wry neck," is a condition characterized by an abnormal, asymmetrical head or neck position. It can be congenital (present at birth) or acquired later in life. Congenital torticollis often arises from muscular issues, such as a tight sternocleidomastoid muscle, which can occur due to positioning in utero or trauma during birth. Acquired torticollis may result from various factors including infections, trauma, or neurological conditions.

The manifestations of torticollis vary but typically include tilting of the head to one side and rotation of the chin toward the opposite side. This can lead to discomfort and functional limitations in neck movement. In infants, it may also affect developmental milestones such as rolling over and crawling.

Anatomical and Muscular Factors Involved in Torticollis

The primary anatomical structure involved in congenital torticollis is the sternocleidomastoid muscle (SCM). The SCM runs from the sternum and clavicle to the mastoid process behind the ear. When this muscle becomes shortened or tight on one side, it causes the head to tilt toward that side while rotating away from it.

In addition to the SCM, other muscles such as the trapezius and splenius capitis can also contribute to neck positioning abnormalities. Understanding these anatomical relationships is crucial for effective treatment planning. For instance, if there are compensatory patterns involving other muscles due to SCM tightness, these must be addressed during intervention.

Effective Assessment Techniques for Accurate Diagnosis

Accurate diagnosis of torticollis involves a comprehensive assessment that includes both clinical evaluation and imaging studies when necessary. Clinicians typically perform a physical examination focusing on:

1. **Range of Motion:** Assessing active and passive range of motion in all directions helps determine the extent of restriction.
2. **Palpation:** Feeling for tightness or asymmetry in neck muscles provides insight into muscular involvement.
3. **Observation:** Noting head posture during various activities can reveal compensatory behaviors.
4. **Neurological Assessment:** Evaluating neurological function ensures that there are no underlying conditions contributing to symptoms.

In some cases, imaging studies like X-rays or MRI may be warranted to rule out structural abnormalities or other pathologies.

Significance of Timely Intervention and Management Strategies

Early intervention is critical for managing torticollis effectively. Delayed treatment can lead to secondary complications such as facial asymmetry, developmental delays, and chronic pain issues later in life. The goals of early intervention include:

1. **Restoring Normal Range of Motion:** Physical therapy techniques such as stretching exercises for the affected muscles are essential.
2. **Strengthening Opposing Muscles:** Strengthening exercises for muscles on the opposite side help restore balance.
3. **Positioning Strategies:** Educating caregivers on proper positioning during feeding and playtime can prevent further tightening.
4. **Surgical Options:** In severe cases where conservative measures fail after 12 months of age, surgical intervention may be considered to release tight muscles.

Timely management not only improves physical outcomes but also enhances overall quality of life by allowing children to engage fully in their developmental activities without restrictions.

In summary, understanding torticollis—its origins, anatomical factors involved, assessment techniques for diagnosis, and significance of early intervention—is vital for effective management strategies that promote optimal outcomes.

Chapter

Understanding Torticollis

Anatomy of the Neck and Sternocleidomastoid Muscle

The human neck is a complex structure that serves as a critical connection between the head and the torso. It comprises several anatomical components, including bones, muscles, nerves, and blood vessels. The cervical vertebrae form the backbone of the neck, providing support and flexibility. The muscles in the neck are responsible for various movements such as rotation, flexion, and extension of the head.

Among these muscles, the sternocleidomastoid (SCM) plays a pivotal role in neck movement and stabilization. The SCM is a paired muscle that extends from two points: the manubrium of the sternum (the upper part of the breastbone) and the clavicle (collarbone). It inserts at the mastoid process, which is located behind the ear on the temporal bone of the skull. This unique positioning allows for significant mobility; when one side of the SCM contracts, it causes rotation of the head to the opposite side while tilting it toward the same side. When both sides contract simultaneously, they work together to flex and extend the neck.

The SCM also has important functional roles beyond movement; it aids in respiration by assisting with inhalation when necessary. Its involvement in various activities makes it susceptible to strain or injury, which can lead to conditions like torticollis.

Types of Torticollis: Congenital vs. Acquired

Torticollis is characterized by an abnormal twisting or tilting of the neck that can result in discomfort or pain. There are two primary types of torticollis: congenital and acquired.

- Congenital Torticollis: This type is typically noticeable at birth or shortly thereafter. Congenital torticollis often arises from trauma during delivery or abnormal positioning during fetal development in utero. For instance, if a baby is positioned in a way that compresses one side of their neck during gestation or experiences physical stress during childbirth (such as shoulder dystocia), this can lead to muscular shortening on one side

13

of their neck. As a result, infants may present with a tilted head posture where they favor one side over another. Treatment usually involves physical therapy aimed at stretching and strengthening exercises to improve range of motion.

- Acquired Torticollis: Unlike congenital torticollis, acquired torticollis develops later in life due to various external factors or underlying health conditions. Common causes include trauma (such as whiplash injuries), infections (like meningitis), muscle spasms due to stress or overuse, or prolonged positioning—such as sleeping on one's side for extended periods without changing positions. In adults, acquired torticollis may also be associated with neurological disorders such as cervical dystonia (a condition characterized by involuntary muscle contractions). Treatment options for acquired torticollis vary depending on its cause but may include physical therapy, medications for pain relief or muscle relaxation, and sometimes surgical interventions if conservative measures fail.

Signs and Symptoms

Symptoms of torticollis can include:

- Uneven positioning of the head and neck.
- Neck pain or stiffness.
- Headaches.
- Limited range of motion in the neck.
- In infants, noticeable flattening on one side of the head due to a consistent tilt.

Uneven Positioning of the Head and Neck

One of the hallmark signs of torticollis is the uneven positioning of the head. This may manifest as a tilt to one side, where the chin points toward one shoulder while the ear on that side is closer to the shoulder. This asymmetry can be noticeable when observing an individual from behind or in profile. In infants, this unevenness may lead to developmental concerns if not addressed promptly.

Neck Pain or Stiffness

Individuals with torticollis often experience pain or stiffness in their neck muscles. This discomfort can range from mild to severe and may worsen with movement. The stiffness is typically due to muscle spasms that occur as a result of the abnormal positioning of the head and neck. Over time, chronic pain can develop if left untreated, leading to further complications such as muscle tightness or weakness.

Headaches

Headaches are another common symptom associated with torticollis. The tension created by the abnormal muscle contractions in the neck can lead to tension-type headaches or even migraines in some individuals. These headaches may be exacerbated by stress or prolonged periods of poor posture, which are often seen in those suffering from torticollis.

Limited Range of Motion in the Neck

A significant limitation in neck mobility is often observed in individuals with torticollis. This restricted range of motion can make it difficult for individuals to turn their heads fully in one direction or look up and down without discomfort. The inability to move freely can impact daily activities such as driving, exercising, or even simple tasks like looking over one's shoulder.

Flattening on One Side of the Head in Infants

In infants diagnosed with congenital torticollis, a noticeable flattening on one side of the head may occur due to consistent tilting towards one side (also known as positional plagiocephaly). This flattening happens because infants spend a lot of time lying on their backs, which can cause pressure on one side of their skull if they consistently favor that position. Early intervention through physical therapy or repositioning techniques is essential to prevent long-term cranial deformities.

Assessment of Torticollis

A thorough physical assessment is crucial for diagnosing and managing torticollis effectively.

Step 1: Patient History Begin the assessment by gathering a comprehensive patient history:

- Onset of Symptoms: Determine when the symptoms began and if they were sudden or gradual.
- Associated Symptoms: Ask about pain, stiffness, or any neurological symptoms such as weakness or numbness.
- Medical History: Inquire about any previous injuries, surgeries, or conditions that may contribute to torticollis.
- Family History: Assess if there is a family history of similar conditions.

Step 2: Observation Conduct a visual inspection of the patient:

- Head Positioning: Observe the position of the head; it may tilt to one side with rotation towards the opposite side.
- Facial Asymmetry: Look for any signs of facial asymmetry which may indicate muscular involvement.
- Posture: Note the overall posture and any compensatory mechanisms used by the patient.

Step 3: Palpation Carefully palpate the neck muscles:

- Muscle Tone: Assess muscle tone in both sternocleidomastoid muscles (SCM) and other surrounding muscles.
- Tenderness: Check for tenderness in affected areas which may indicate muscle strain or spasm.
- Masses or Nodules: Feel for any abnormal masses that could suggest underlying pathology.

Step 4: Range of Motion (ROM) Assessment Evaluate the range of motion in the cervical spine:

- Active ROM Testing: Ask the patient to move their head in all directions (flexion, extension, lateral flexion, and rotation). Note any limitations or pain during these movements.
- Passive ROM Testing: Gently assist with movements to determine if restrictions are due to muscle tightness or joint issues.

Step 5: Neurological Examination Perform a basic neurological examination:

- Reflexes: Test deep tendon reflexes in upper extremities to rule out neurological involvement.
- Sensory Examination: Check for sensory deficits in arms and hands which could indicate nerve compression.

Step 6: Functional Assessment Assess how torticollis affects daily activities:

- Activities of Daily Living (ADLs): Evaluate how neck positioning impacts tasks like eating, grooming, and driving.
- Quality of Life Measures: Use standardized questionnaires if available to assess impact on quality of life.

Step 7: Imaging Studies (if necessary) If indicated based on findings from physical assessment:

- Consider ordering imaging studies such as X-rays or MRI to evaluate structural abnormalities contributing to torticollis.

Importance of Early Detection

The early detection of torticollis can dramatically impact treatment outcomes. Implementing—and adhering to—an effective treatment plan promotes muscle rehabilitation and normalization of neck positioning the sooner it is initiated. Ideally, this enables both children and adults to regain and maintain an appropriate range of motion, improving their overall quality of

Impact of Early Detection The early detection of torticollis is crucial for several reasons:

1. **Timely Intervention**: Identifying torticollis at an early stage allows for prompt intervention. This is vital because the earlier treatment begins, the more effective it tends to be. Early intervention can prevent the development of compensatory postures and secondary musculoskeletal issues that may arise if left untreated.

2. **Muscle Rehabilitation**: Early detection facilitates targeted rehabilitation strategies aimed at stretching and strengthening the affected muscles. Physical therapy is often employed as a primary treatment modality, focusing on exercises that promote muscle balance and flexibility. When initiated early, these interventions can lead to significant improvements in muscle function.

3. **Normalization of Neck Positioning**: With timely treatment, individuals with torticollis can achieve normalization of neck positioning. This not only alleviates discomfort but also enhances overall mobility and functionality. Proper alignment reduces strain on surrounding muscles and joints, contributing to better posture and reducing the risk of future complications.

4. **Improved Range of Motion**: One of the primary goals of treating torticollis is to restore a full range of motion in the neck. Early detection allows for consistent therapeutic exercises that can help regain this range more effectively than if treatment were delayed.

5. **Quality of Life Enhancements**: For both children and adults suffering from torticollis, early detection leads to improved quality of life outcomes. Individuals are less likely to experience pain or discomfort associated with restricted movement, which can enhance daily activities such as playing for children or work-related tasks for adults.

6. **Psychosocial Benefits**: In children particularly, having a visible condition like torticollis can lead to social stigma or psychological distress due to differences in appearance or mobility compared to peers. Early intervention helps mitigate these effects by promoting normal development and social interactions.
7. **Long-term Outcomes**: Studies have shown that individuals who receive early treatment for torticollis tend to have better long-term outcomes regarding neck function and overall physical health compared to those who begin treatment later in life.

Chapter

"Effective Techniques, Exercises, and Environmental Adaptations for Managing Torticollis in Children"

Treatment Protocol Should Include:

1. Massage
2. Passive and Active Range of Motion
3. Strengthening Exercises
4. Positioning and Handling Guidelines
5. Visual Exercises
6. Righting Reactions/Postural Education
7. Environmental Adaptations

Massage

- Begin with gentle massage.
- Run fingers along muscle belly and press thumbs gently into tight spots along sternocleidomastoid muscle.

  Goals: Reduce tightness of muscle, increase flexibility and range of motion.

How to Perform a Gentle Massage on the Sternocleidomastoid Muscle

Step 1: Preparation

- Find a comfortable and quiet space where you can focus on the massage. Ensure that you are seated or lying down in a position that allows easy access to your neck.
- You may want to use a small amount of massage oil or lotion to reduce friction on the skin, but this is optional.

Step 2: Locate the Sternocleidomastoid Muscle

- The sternocleidomastoid (SCM) muscle runs from behind your ear down to your collarbone and breastbone. To locate it, turn your head slightly to one side; you will see the muscle bulging out on the side of your neck.

Step 3: Begin with Gentle Massage

- Start by using your fingertips to gently stroke along the length of the SCM muscle. Use light pressure and move from the base of the skull down towards the collarbone.
- This initial gentle massage helps warm up the muscle and prepares it for deeper work.

Step 4: Apply Pressure with Thumbs

- After warming up, use your thumbs to apply gentle pressure into any tight spots you feel along the muscle belly.
- Focus on areas that feel particularly tense or knotted. Press firmly but avoid causing pain; you should feel a release rather than discomfort.

Step 5: Work on Tight Spots

- Spend extra time on these tight spots, applying pressure for about 15-30 seconds at a time. You can also make small circular motions with your thumbs while maintaining pressure.
- If you find an area that feels especially tight, hold steady pressure there until you feel it begin to relax.

Step 6: Stretching

- After massaging, gently stretch the SCM muscle by tilting your head towards one shoulder while keeping your shoulders relaxed. Hold this position for about 15 seconds and then switch sides.
- This stretching helps increase flexibility and range of motion after releasing tension through massage.

Passive Range of Motion

- Address Head Rotation and Lateral Flexion
- Target the range of motion of child's head and neck.
- Can begin range of motion exercises with a little gentle lateral flexion.

    Goals: To open up the joint space, allow child to more freely move head, reduce range of motion limitations.

Rotation (chin to shoulder)

- Place your one hand on child's shoulder, cup child's head with other hand.
- Slowly turn child's head bringing chin to shoulder.
- Hold this stretch for 10-15 seconds.
- Gradually increase duration of stretch to child's comfort level and tolerance.

Side-Bending (ear to shoulder)

- With child positioned comfortably on his or her back, either on softly padded floor or therapist/caregiver's lap, begin tilting the head to opposite side.
- If you are trying to stretch the muscles on the left side, place your right hand on the child's left shoulder.
- Press down as you use your left hand to tilt the child's right ear to his or her right shoulder.
- Hold this stretch for 10-15 seconds.
- Gradually increase duration of stretch to child's comfort level and tolerance.

Shoulder Depression

- Provide downward pressure at shoulders.

    Goals: To open up joint space, decrease elevation of shoulders, reduce muscle tightness.

Lower Trunk Rotation (guided rolling)

- Using pelvis to guide from supine into side lying to prone on both sides.
- Begin by building momentum with gentle rocking side to side.

- As child gains mastery your handling will decrease, as child is able to roll independently.

Goals: Promote transitional movements, encourage symmetry in rolling, and activation of both sides of body.

Strengthening Exercises

- Targeting muscles of head/neck, trunk, back and upper extremities.
- Be mindful of strength imbalance and compensations as you perform these activities.

Exercises on Therapy Ball

- Practice tummy time on therapy ball.
- While supporting child at trunk, gently rock side to side and front to back.
- You can place mirror in front of child to promote alignment as well.

- Practice therapy ball work with child seated to promote trunk strength and stability.
- Allowing child to lean back and promote rotation to return to upward seated posture.
- Lower support as child becomes stronger.

Exercises on Tummy Time Pillow or Incline Ramp

- Encourage head/neck extension and rotation.
- Also facilitates upper body weight bearing.

Positioning for Torticollis Treatment

Prone (or Tummy Down position)

- Encourage "tummy time" by placing child on stomach.
- Slowly increase duration as child builds strength and tolerance for longer intervals.

- Using tummy time mirror, fun toy, or even your child's favourite pet (pictured above Abe and Daze gaze longingly into each other's eyes!).
- Encourage child to look away from restricted side.

    Goals: Encourage head, neck and upper body strength, facilitate pushing off surface, vertical visual gaze, promote fluid head rotation and range of motion!

- Can place child on soft incline wedge or with small towel or swaddle blanket rolled up under child's chest.
- Position arms over the bolster with hands or forearms contacting surface.

- Encourage weight bearing through arms, by gently supporting under arms to facilitate lifting upper body off surface.
- Another great way to practice tummy time, especially in children who are more reluctant, is to place child tummy to tummy on you.

Sidelying (or Child Positioned on Side)

- Encourage side lying so that head and neck are turned away from restricted side, can utilise rolled up towel or pillow to position.
- Keep child engaged in this position and allow them to utilise both right and left arms in play.

In Carseat/Stroller

- Encourage midline using supportive headrest or infant support as pictured

In Carrier

- Encourage in-facing position until baby has head control and ability to right themselves and orient to both sides.
- Can promote looking away from area of restriction during time in carrier.
- One of our favourite carriers is the Beco Gemini Carrier, as pictured above!

Handling for Torticollis Treatment

Sidelying Carry

- Carry child with one arm positioned under area of restriction to facilitate stretch and encourage child to look away from limited side.

Superman Hold

- Supporting child in order to encourage extended position (can be done in arms or on lap).

Visual Exercises for Torticollis Treatment

Visual Tracking

- Promote tracking with fluid eye movements to both right and left sides.
- Stimulating visual or auditory objects may help motivate.
- Encourage visual tracking in all developmental positions: supine, side lying, prone, quadruped, supported sitting.

Exercises for Improving Visual Tracking

Tracking Objects Side to Side

- **Setup:** Use a brightly colored toy or an object that makes noise.
- **Execution:** Hold the toy at eye level and slowly move it from one side to the other, encouraging your child to turn their head and follow the object with their eyes. Start by moving it towards the non-preferred side (the side they do not naturally turn towards) to promote movement in that direction.
- **Duration:** Repeat this exercise for 5-10 minutes, allowing breaks as needed.

Vertical Tracking

- **Setup:** Use a hanging mobile or a toy that can be moved up and down.

- **Execution:** Position the mobile above your child's head and gently move it up and down. Encourage your child to look up and down, following the movement with their eyes while keeping their head still.
- **Duration:** Perform this exercise for about 5-10 minutes.

Mirror Play

- **Setup:** Place a mirror in front of your child during tummy time or when they are sitting.
- **Execution:** Encourage your child to look at themselves in the mirror while you hold toys on either side of them. This will encourage them to turn their head and track objects visually as they see themselves move.
- **Duration:** Engage in this activity for 10-15 minutes daily.

Obstacle Course

- **Setup:** Create a simple obstacle course using pillows, toys, or soft blocks.
- **Execution:** As your child navigates through the course, place toys at various angles that require them to turn their heads and track visually as they reach for them.
- **Duration:** Spend about 15-20 minutes playing through the course.

Interactive Games

- **Setup:** Use games that involve movement, such as rolling a ball back and forth.
- **Execution:** Sit facing your child and roll a ball towards them while encouraging them to watch its path closely. You can also use different colored balls or sound-making balls to keep their attention focused on tracking.
- **Duration:** Play these interactive games for 10-15 minutes.

Incorporating Visual Tracking into Daily Activities Integrate visual tracking exercises into daily routines by encouraging activities like reading books together where characters move across pages or watching videos where objects move across the screen. This helps reinforce visual skills while making it enjoyable for your child.

Righting Reactions/Postural Education

Weight Shifting on Therapy Ball

- Weight shifting via ball in supine/prone/supported sitting.

Postural Education on Dynamic Surface (Dyna-disc or Incline wedge)

- Using dyna-disc or incline wedge to challenge trunk strength/stability in sitting and shoulder strength/stability in prone propping.

Environmental Adaptations for Torticollis Treatment

1. Position child in the crib or on changing table to encourage looking away from restriction, place visually stimulating objects on opposite side of room.
2. Position toys away from restriction to encourage child to look and reach with upper extremity away from affected side.
3. While bottle or breast feeding, position child to stretch restricted side, alternate regularly.
4. Use mirror during side lying play to encourage gaze.
5. When picking child up from floor, crib or changing table, facilitate roll to one side and then lift up, alternate regularly.

Clinical Case Study of Torticollis

Patient Profile

- **Name**: Emily
- **Age:** 6 months
- **Gender**: Female
- **Medical History**: No significant medical history; born full-term via vaginal delivery.
- **Presenting Complaint**: Parents report that Emily's head tilts to the right side and she prefers to look left. They noticed this tilt shortly after birth.

Assessment

1. **Observation:**
   - Head tilt to the right with rotation towards the left.
   - Limited range of motion in cervical spine when attempting to turn head to the right.

2. **Palpation:**
   - Tightness noted in the right SCM muscle.
   - No palpable masses or abnormalities in other cervical muscles.

3. **Range of Motion (ROM) Testing:**
   - Active ROM: Limited right rotation (approximately 30 degrees compared to 70 degrees on the left).
   - Passive ROM: Slightly better than active but still limited on the right side.

4. **Functional Assessment:**
   - Difficulty in visual tracking towards the right side.
   - Preference for turning head left during playtime.

5. **Diagnosis:**
   - Congenital muscular torticollis confirmed based on clinical findings and history.

Treatment Plan

1. **Goals:**
   - Improve range of motion in cervical spine.
   - Decrease muscle tightness in SCM.
   - Promote symmetrical head positioning.
   - Educate parents on home exercises and positioning strategies.

2. **Interventions:**

a. Stretching Exercises:

   - Gentle stretching of the right SCM muscle performed daily, holding each stretch for 15-30 seconds, repeated 3 times per session.
   - Encourage passive lateral flexion towards the left side while stabilizing the shoulder girdle.

b. Strengthening Exercises:

- Strengthening exercises for neck extensors and contralateral SCM initiated once flexibility improves.
- Activities such as tummy time to promote overall neck strength and stability.

c. Positioning Techniques:

- Advise parents on positioning Emily during feeding and playtime to encourage looking towards her right side.
- Use toys placed on her right side to stimulate visual tracking and encourage head movement.

3. **Frequency of Treatment:**
   - Bi-weekly physiotherapy sessions for 8 weeks, with reassessment at each visit.

Progress Monitoring

After four weeks of treatment:

1. **Reassessment Findings:**
   - Improved active ROM with increased right rotation (now approximately 50 degrees).
   - Decreased tightness noted upon palpation of SCM.
2. **Functional Improvements:**
   - Increased ability to visually track objects placed on her right side.
   - Parents report less preference for turning head left during activities.
3. **Adjustment of Treatment Plan:** Based on progress, continue stretching and strengthening exercises while introducing more dynamic movements like reaching for toys from different angles.

Outcome

At eight weeks post-initiation of therapy:

1. Full range of motion achieved with no observable head tilt during static observation.

2. Parents educated about ongoing home exercise programs to maintain gains achieved through therapy.
3. Follow-up scheduled at six months post-treatment for monitoring any potential recurrence or need for further intervention.

Conclusion

This case study illustrates a successful approach to managing congenital torticollis through targeted physiotherapy interventions focusing on stretching, strengthening, and functional activities tailored specifically for pediatric patients.

Conclusion

Torticollis, while challenging, is a condition that can be effectively managed and treated with early intervention and appropriate care. Understanding its nuances, causes, risk factors, and techniques for assessment equips both healthcare providers and patients with the knowledge necessary for safeguarding neck health and ensuring a better quality of life.

Reference

1. Cristea, F., Ichim, P., Gheorghiu, A., & Jos, D.D. (2018). Kinetotheray in Torticollis to Child. The Annals of "Dunarea de Jos" University of Galati. Fascicle XV, Physical Education and Sport Management.
2. Tomczak, K., & Rosman, N. (2013). Torticollis. *Journal of Child Neurology, 28*, 365 - 378.
3. Robert N. Hensinger, Eric T. Jones *Developmental Medicine & Child Neurology,* 1982
4. Searls YR, Dugas JR, Loder RT, Frick SL. "Congenital Muscular Torticollis: Current Concepts and Review of Treatment." Journal of Pediatric Orthopaedics. This review could provide a more modern understanding of treatment strategies.
5. Cranial Remolding Therapy Guidelines—these guidelines could be important if discussing plagiocephaly associated with torticollis.
6. APTA's Pediatric Section Publications—they may have updated handbooks or case studies focusing on physical therapy for pediatric torticollis.
7. Coulter-O'Berry C, et al., "Effectiveness of Physical Therapy Interventions for Infants With Congenital Muscular Torticollis: A Systematic Review." Pediatric Physical Therapy Journal. This study will give you more recent data on intervention efficacy
8. https://www.nationwidechildrens.org/family-resources-education/health-wellness-and-safety-resources/helping-hands/exercises-left-torticollis-positioning-for-play
9. Dayasiri, K., & Rao, S. (2021). Fifteen-minute consultation: Evaluation of paediatric torticollis. *Archives of Disease in Childhood, 108*, 17 - 21.

Acknowledgment

I would like to express my sincere gratitude to all the healthcare professionals, researchers, and institutions that have contributed to the understanding and treatment of torticollis. Special thanks to my colleagues for their invaluable insights and support throughout this project. Their expertise has been instrumental in shaping this guide.

Summary

Torticollis, or wry neck, is a condition characterized by an abnormal twisting or tilting of the neck, often noticeable in infants between 4 to 8 weeks of age. Early intervention is critical, as it can prevent complications such as facial asymmetry and limited range of motion. This guide outlines comprehensive treatment protocols, including massage therapy, range of motion exercises, strengthening techniques, and positioning strategies to promote recovery. Effective assessment methods are emphasized to ensure timely diagnosis and management. By understanding the complexities of torticollis, healthcare providers can significantly enhance patient outcomes.

Glossary

- **Torticollis**: A condition involving abnormal positioning of the head and neck, often leading to a tilted or twisted appearance.
- **Sternocleidomastoid Muscle**: A major neck muscle that helps with head rotation and tilting.
- **Congenital Torticollis**: A form of torticollis present at birth, usually due to muscular issues.
- **Acquired Torticollis**: Torticollis that develops later in life due to trauma or underlying health conditions.
- **Range of Motion (ROM)**: The full movement potential of a joint, typically measured in degrees.
- **Massage Therapy**: A treatment technique involving manipulation of muscles to relieve tension and improve flexibility.
- **Visual Tracking**: The ability to follow moving objects with the eyes, important for developmental milestones in children.